Travel 911

Travel 911
A HEALTH GUIDE FOR ADVENTURERS

Yvette McQueen, MD

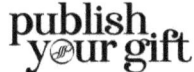

TRAVEL 911
Copyright © 2021 Yvette McQueen
All rights reserved.

Published by Publish Your Gift®
An imprint of Purposely Created Publishing Group, LLC

No part of this book may be reproduced, distributed or transmitted in any form by any means, graphic, electronic, or mechanical, including photocopy, recording, taping, or by any information storage or retrieval system, without permission in writing from the publisher, except in the case of reprints in the context of reviews, quotes, or references.

Printed in the United States of America

ISBN: 978-1-64484-393-2 (print)
ISBN: 978-1-64484-394-9 (ebook)

Photo Credits: Adobe Stock Photography Licensed
CPR and AED Algorithm created by Yvette McQueen, MD

Disclaimer: Segments of the written word have previously been used in lectures, published in blogs and social media articles, and/or are taken from *Travelpedia: A Quick Guide on How to Travel Efficiently, Healthy and Safely*, all materials written by the author.

Special discounts are available on bulk quantity purchases by book clubs, associations and special interest groups. For details email: sales@publishyourgift.com or call (888) 949-6228.
For information log on to www.PublishYourGift.com

Table of Contents

Introduction vii

Chapter 1: Health Items to Pack for Travel
& Basics to Healthy Travel 1

Chapter 2: Jet Lag 11

Chapter 3: Blood Clots 17

Chapter 4: Traveler's Diarrhea 21

Chapter 5: Fever & Malaria 27

Chapter 6: Water Accidents & Illnesses 31

Chapter 7: Altitude Sickness & Motion
Sickness 35

Chapter 8: Environmental Problems 41

Chapter 9: Skin Problems 51

Chapter 10: Prevention & Medical Travel
Insurance 61

Chapter 11: First Aid as a Non-Medical
Traveler – Accidents, Cuts, and Recognizing
a Medical Emergency 67

Chapter 12: Post-Travel Illnesses 79

Appendix 85

About the Author 95

Hello Fellow Travelers,

You are all ready to set out on an adventure, vacation, and/or a few days of fun. You have planned and paid for your experience, but the one thing you probably didn't plan for is sickness and emergencies. Unfortunately, those incidents sometimes interfere with the best organized plans. As an Emergency Medicine doctor, I always keep in the back of my mind the unfortunate possibilities and pack extra for those events. I wanted to share with my fellow spirit adventurers and world travelers how to avoid disruption in your experience. This guide gives you information on items to pack, situations to anticipate, and how to recognize/handle a medical emergency as a non-medical person. Carry it with you on all your travels.

Travel well!
Yvette McQueen, MD

Chapter 1

Health Items to Pack for Travel & Basics to Healthy Travel

You are ready for your vacation, business trip, or general travel. You should include health-related and priority items on your packing list. You can adjust the items according to the type of traveling you are doing: relaxation, adventure, mission, etc.

On every trip, you should take a mini first aid kit which includes Band-Aids, wound cleanser, and antibiotic ointment. As you progress to different travels, you will add bandages, ace wraps, eye wash, and other items. Here is a list of other appropriate health-related items to remember:

1. Medications (Over-the-counter and prescriptions) – Do not pack these in the checked luggage. If you are traveling internationally, take your prescription medications in the

original bottles with your name on them. In some countries, the daily pill boxes with unnamed pills are not allowed when going through customs. Check with the country to see if they will allow or ban certain psychiatric and enhancement medications. Take your favorite over-the-counter medications for pain, fever, or allergies; you may not find them where you are going, or they may have different names in another language. If your medication is an injection and needles are required, please pack them together.

2. Equipment – Take any medical equipment you need for survival (oxygen, CPAP, peritoneal dialysis), and you should have a physician's letter stating these items are necessary. Also, take instructions for the equipment in case someone other than you needs to operate it.

3. First aid items – bandages, alcohol swabs, wound cleanser, antibiotic ointment

4. Allergy (medications for environment allergies and allergic reactions) – If you know you have an allergy to certain foods or insects, please carry an EpiPen for

emergencies. And once again, if traveling internationally, a doctor's letter should accompany the EpiPen.

MEDICATIONS TO TAKE WHILE TRAVELING

- Pain and fever relief
- Anti-diarrhea
- Motion or sea sickness
- Altitude sickness
- Antihistamine or allergy
- Anti-acid
- Decongestant
- Cough drops or cough suppressant (non-liquid)
- Laxative

PREVENTIVE ITEMS

- Facial mask
- Mosquito or insect repellent
- Hand sanitizer and wipes
- Antiseptic wipes
- Sunscreen

- Aloe
- Water purification tablets

FIRST AID

- Hydrocortisone or allergy cream
- Antiseptic wound cleanser
- Antibacterial ointment
- Aloe
- Eye drops
- Band-Aids
- Elastic bandage or ace wrap
- Oral rehydration tablets/salts
- Disposable gloves

THE BASICS OF HEALTHY TRAVEL

Traveling is a way we balance our lives, but frequent traveling can take a toll on your body, eating habits, and overall wellness. The hustle of getting on trains and planes, the packing and organization, or co-ordinating family or friends increases the stress of your adventure. And of course, the change of time zones and sleeping habitats affect your equilibrium.

Travel 911

It is essential to incorporate daily wellness into your life to maintain a steady rhythm and reduce the stress on your body. By incorporating wellness behaviors in your travel, you can achieve an overall superb quality of life as a traveler.

1. Hydration is an important aspect of your travel health. Flying will dehydrate you; the recycled air in the cabin, the altitude, the pressurized compartment, and changes in your daily routine all contribute to this factor. People also do not drink as much water before a flight because they don't want to get up and use the closet bathroom as often.

   However, hydration keeps your blood circulating, reduces risks of blood clots, reduces jet lag, lubricates your joints, and improves your overall health. You cannot bring liquids through airport security, but you can bring an empty bottle, reusable bottle/canister, or a collapsible travel bottle. Airports now have filling stations for you to refill the bottles with filtered water rather than having to pay two to five dollars per bottle.

   For an average adult, daily hydration maintenance should be half of his or her body weight in ounces. Example: body weight of 150 pounds = 75 ounces of water. A hydration test of adequacy is tenting of the skin on the back of the hand. Pinch the back of the hand and if the skin flattens immediately, you are adequately hydrated. If it does not, then consider drinking more water. A dry mouth is a late sign of dehydration. Fluids that can be used to rehydrate are water, coconut water, or 2 percent milk. Excessive sweating and diarrhea resulting in fluid loss requires replacement. Water and electrolyte replacement can be done with this formula: one to two cups of water + juice from half a squeezed lemon + one-fourth teaspoon sea salt + two teaspoons honey. If you are on a water restriction, please consult with your physician about your daily water intake.

2. Physical wellness is the need for keeping the body healthy and physically active. During travel, consider keeping your normal eating routine and times because your body likes a schedule. As you are arranging travel activities, consider ones that include walking tours, biking, or other active adventures.

3. Boost your immune system by getting enough sleep. Sleep is the time for the body to repair daily. The average sleep needed is seven to eight hours for adults and ten to twelve hours for children each night. Do not stay up the night before you travel; you may not be able to sleep in the car, train, or plane as expected. If you have trouble sleeping, there are over-the-counter sleep aids such as melatonin; consult with your physician before taking extra medications and supplements. Adjust your sleep pattern according to the time zone of your destination. Also, consider taking daily vitamins to compliment your immune system.

4. Planning, anticipation, time schedule, and traveling companions can create stressful emotions. Your immune system is affected severely by your stress levels. You can reduce your travel stress with adequate sleep, relaxing during delays by reading or an activity you enjoy, and napping in between tours. Time and task management techniques help you organize and enjoy stress-free travel.

5. Keep your energy up. Avoid foods with high sugar; these only provide temporary energy and will make you fatigued later. Protein snacks and nuts (if you don't have an allergy) are a good afternoon source of energy to keep you going while traversing the city.

6. Wash your hands often. Soap and water are the best way to prevent transmitting germs to yourself. You should use warm water with soapy suds to wash both hands. Wash for at least twenty seconds and make sure you get in between the fingers.

7. Keep hand sanitizer and antiseptic wipes with you. Hand sanitizer is the next best solution when soap and water is not available. Place it on both hands, rub them together, and allow them to air dry for fifteen seconds. People transfer germs and viruses when their hands touch objects, and then they touch their faces. Viruses can live eight to twelve hours on an object.

8. Places to use antiseptic wipes: airplane seat armrests, seat buttons, screens, and tray tables. Likewise, also use antiseptic wipes on

rental car steering wheels, gear shift, knobs, buttons, door handles, keys, and key fob. When you arrive at your hotel or lodging site, use wipes on hotel room door handles, light switches, lamp switches, TV remote, telephone, and baby changing stations.

9. Facial masks, whether reusable cloth or disposable (3-ply), are recommended and mandated in some countries for travel since March 2020. Proper wearing of a facial mask includes covering the nose and mouth. It should be worn during travel in public areas and social gatherings to avoid transmitting and obtaining the respiratory virus SARS-CoV2.

The next few chapters will describe common travel health problems, prevention, self-treatment, and when to seek professional medical help.

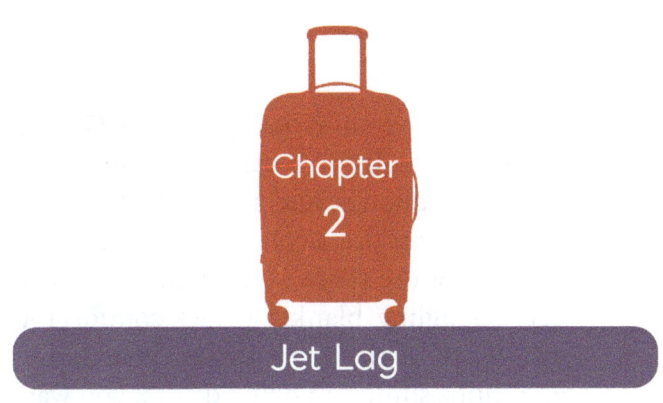

Chapter 2

Jet Lag

If you fly and change to a time zone that is a three or more hours difference than the time zone you live in, you may experience jet lag. You land feeling sluggish and fatigued; this feeling may last up to twenty-four hours after landing. The change of time zones and extensive traveling throws off the circadian rhythm (your internal time clock) in your body for a while.

Jet lag will cause insomnia, excessive daytime fatigue, irritability, impaired judgment and performance, and the inability to concentrate.

You may avoid it by following these tips:

1. Get rest the night before. Do not stay up packing or partying the night before with the expectation of getting sleep on the airplane. You may not be able to sleep, or you may be stuck in a middle seat or in a row

with an active child or crying baby (It's not the baby's fault). Use ear plugs, noise-cancelling earphones, and an eye shade to help you sleep on the airplane. And use a personal (not the reused ones that airlines offer) snuggling blanket to get comfortable rest. Lack of sleep can impair your brain's functions similar to being drunk; you want to be aware and functional when you reach your destination.

Transition your hourly clock a few days before you travel to the new time zone. At least forty-eight to seventy-two hours before your trip, try to function in the destination's time zone, a gradual change of two to three-hour difference. Once arriving at your destination, expose yourself to sunlight to help you adjust. Most flights that leave from the east coast to Europe leave at night; you'll arrive at your destination between 6:00 a.m. to 9:00 a.m. Most European hotels will accommodate the traveler and have some rooms available for early arrivals. You can always call the hotel one to two days prior to arrival to arrange for early arrival. When you land at your destination during the morning or daytime, do not go to sleep. If your hotel room is available, take a hot, rejuvenating shower. If the room is not ready, store your luggage at your lodging, then hit the streets and follow the local time. Have an early dinner and then bedtime.

2. Stay hydrated with water! Flying and travel will cause dehydration since your normal routine is changed. So, hydrate before you travel, during the flight, and after the flight. Yes, the water will cause you to go to the bathroom more, but it helps with the circulation in your legs and reduces the risk of blood clots. The true test of hydration is the color of your urine: pale yellow, clear, and see-through means good hydration.

3. Eat light. Heavy foods, high carbohydrates, and fried foods will cause fatigue and sleepiness. High sodium foods will cause water retention and leg swelling. In addition, gas-producing foods, including bubbly or carbonated drinks, expand in the pressurized airplane setting, causing abdominal bloating and discomfort. Avoid these foods

at least twenty-four hours before the flight or else you may feel like you instantly gained ten pounds mid-flight.

4. Foods that can cause gas include: broccoli, cabbage, cauliflower, beans, lentils, apples, fluffy wheat, oats, onions, corn, potatoes, pears, peaches, milk, and soft cheese. Try to eat meals during the normal mealtimes of your destination; when you land your breakfast may be their dinner meal time.

5. Limit caffeinated and alcoholic beverages. These also contribute to dehydration. These are stimulants. They will keep you awake and active but will only add to jet lag and may cause insomnia.

6. Wear loose comfortable clothing or clothes that allow moisture wicking (absorb sweat and moisture away from the body). I wear clothes made of breathable material (cotton, linen, rayon) in case of sweating. Layer your clothing for on and off versatility due to climate changes and the cold airplane.

7. Walk and stay active to increase circulation. You should move every two hours while awake on the airplane. Once you get to your destination, be sure to take a twenty-minute

walk after eating a meal to maintain consistent digestive health and regularity.

8. Grounding is not scientific but promoted by wellness theory. You need to kick off your shoes and walk barefoot (safely) on the ground of your current time zone. Touch the grass, sand, mud, or concrete with your toes/feet. Grounding connects your body to the earth of the destination.

9. A natural supplement like the hormone melatonin regulates the circadian rhythm. It helps to reduce jet lag symptoms and helps with sleep. Please consult with your personal physician before taking supplements and medications.

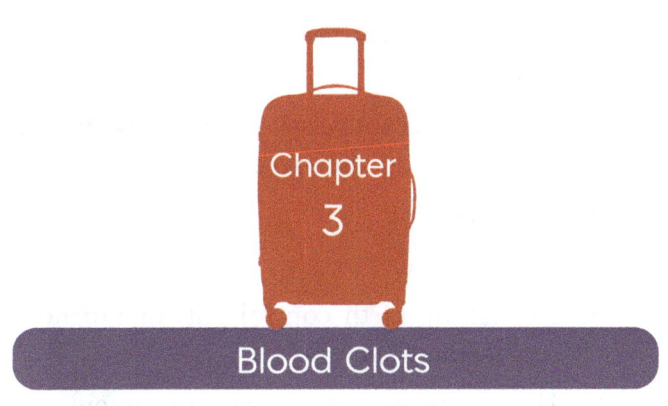

Blood Clots

Blood clots can be deadly and should be taken very seriously. When you travel via car, train, or plane for longer than four hours, you increase your risk of developing blood clots, also known as deep vein thrombosis and pulmonary embolism (DVT/PE). Blood clots form when you are not moving for a long time. The blood in the veins is thick and becomes sluggish. DVT is when a blood clot forms in the leg, and the most common location is the lower leg. Blood clots may travel to your lungs. These are called pulmonary emboli (PE), a condition that will decrease your oxygen levels, strain your heart, and can cause death. If this occurs, seek medical treatment immediately.

You are at increased risk for DVT/PE if you:

1. Have had DVT/PE in the past

2. Have had recent surgery (especially abdominal or orthopedic surgery)
3. Are pregnant
4. Are a smoker
5. Are taking birth control pills or hormone replacement therapy
6. Have cancer, restricted movement, or blood-clotting problems
7. Have a family history of DVT/PE
8. Are obese
9. Have recently broken a bone
10. Frequent fliers and/or in the flight industry

If you have any of these conditions, talk to your doctor before traveling. People at higher risk for DVT/PE may be prescribed medication during travel.

The signs and symptoms of blood clots show up as pain, cough, difficulty breathing, or sometimes a mild fever.

A DVT will cause calf pain in the lower leg usually one more than the other. One leg may be more swollen than the other (two to three times its normal size), skin is hot to the touch, calves hurt to touch, redness exists, and there is pain with foot and toe movement or raising your toes.

Blood clots or pulmonary emboli (PE) in the lungs show up as chest pain, sharp pain with taking a deep breath, difficulty breathing or catching your breath, breathing fast, shallow breaths, sometimes fever, and low oxygenation when tested. There may possibly be a persistent cough.

To reduce risk and prevent DVT/PE during flights:

1. Stay hydrated – It keeps the blood flowing and you moving by going to the bathroom.
2. Wear loose-fitting clothing.
3. Walk around every two hours. Exercise and stretch your legs and arms at least once an hour. Pump your legs up and down, stretching the calves. While sitting, perform toe touches/tip toe crunches and move your feet up and down. You may also stand and march in place.
4. Wear compression socks or stockings that reduce leg swelling and encourage blood flow.

5. If physician approved, some people take aspirin or other blood thinners.

If you have a concern or suspect that you have blood clots with leg swelling, leg pain, chest pain and/or difficulty breathing, seek medical attention immediately. Go to the nearest hospital or emergency department. A range of tests which cannot be done in a doctor's office including a simple blood test, an ultrasound, and/or CT scan of the chest are necessary to rule out blood clots.

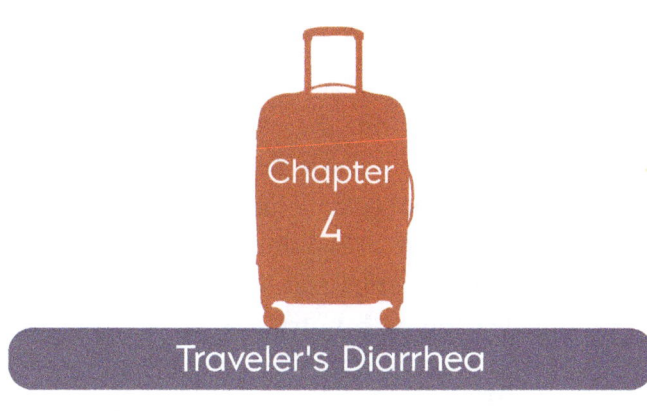

Chapter 4

Traveler's Diarrhea

Diarrhea is the most common illness associated with travel. The definition of diarrhea is determined by the number of stools, three or more unformed stools in a twenty-four hour period. The medical professional will diagnose the cause by the appearance, smell, blood in the stool, or associated fever. Traveler's diarrhea can be caused by bacteria (E. coli, Campylobacter, Salmonella) from water or food ingestion, a virus (norovirus, rotavirus) spread by person to person contact, or a parasite (Giardia) through water contact. So poor hygiene, lack of handwashing, contaminated foods/water, poor cooking preparations, and raw food puts you at risk of developing it.

Persistent diarrhea can cause obstruction of the intestine and/or dehydration, since the intestines are pulling water out of your tissues and blood, attempting to wash out the bacteria. Accompanying symptoms may include nausea, vomiting, loss of appetite, headache, and fatigue. Children and the elderly are more at risk for severe dehydration that may require hospitalization.

Many developing countries of the world do not have clean water sources. You may be in an area that uses a community water source from a river or lake. That water is not only used for drinking but also for bathing, watering the animals, and washing clothes. You can easily be exposed to several bacteria and/or parasites. Your gastrointestinal system is not immune to the local bacteria; therefore, you develop diarrhea and lose a large quantity of your body's water.

If you are unsure of the water source, use bottled water for drinking and cooking.

When eating in a developing country, boil it, cook it, peel it, or forget it!

You are no longer in the US, and the Food and Drug Administration (FDA) guidelines regarding food preparation and storage no longer apply. In many countries, you will find open air markets with the daily meats and produce on display without any methods of preservation.

Unclean water and food can cause food poisoning and diarrhea but also other more serious diseases such as hepatitis A or typhoid. The CDC has an app called "Can I Eat This?" that you can download for free to help with your international journey.

Other points to keep in mind:

- Eat cooked food while it is hot. Avoid eating food that has been sitting out for a while.
- Eat fruits and vegetables only if you can peel them or wash them with clean water. Therefore, salads and salsa should be avoided.
- Avoid raw meat and "bush" meat (game meat of non-domesticated animals). The source of the meat is unknown and typically a wild animal; your body is not used to processing it.
- Avoid raw or runny eggs.
- Use bottled water for drinking and cooking. Coffee and tea must be steaming hot before it is consumed. Tap water can be treated with chlorine or purification tablets or disinfected by boiling. Most five and four-star hotels have water filtration

systems but contact the staff to find out about their water sources.

- According to the CDC, "Drink only water, sodas, or sports drinks that are canned or bottled and sealed (carbonated is safer because the bubbles indicate that it was sealed at the factory)." Avoid ice in drinks. It was most likely made with the local tap water.

- Pasteurized milk from a sealed bottle is fine but be careful of milk or cream sitting in an open container. People with compromised immune systems and pregnant women must avoid unpasteurized milk and dairy products (cheese, yogurts, etc.).

But you can develop traveler's diarrhea in the USA also; campsite creeks/rivers are a source of bacteria and parasites as are raw/contaminated seafood and uncooked meat from diseased animals.

Dehydration is a major complication in a traveler with diarrhea. To avoid dehydration with diarrhea, drink eight ounces of water every time you have a bowel movement.

If you develop diarrhea, drink eight to ten ounces of fluid (250 ml) with each stool. Fluid replacement can be bottled water, rehydration/electrolyte fluids, coconut water, or 2 percent milk. If the diarrhea persists more than forty-eight hours, seek medical help, particularly if you are very young, a senior citizen, or a person with a chronic disease.

***

Side Note: Contaminated water in developing countries also can affect your grooming, bathing, and swimming. Beware of cuts or open wounds, no matter how small, on your body; they must be covered, and you should avoid contact with the water. This includes cuts you get while shaving that you then rinse with the water. Use filtered or bottled water to clean wounds, wash your face after shaving, and brushing your teeth. Do not swallow the water while taking a shower. Wear sandals or flip-flops while taking a shower in case the drainage system is slow and the water pools on the shower floor. Parasites and worms can enter your body from the water through your feet. Do not swim in cloudy water. Some bacteria can be inhaled by steam or vapors in steam baths or while using a hookah.

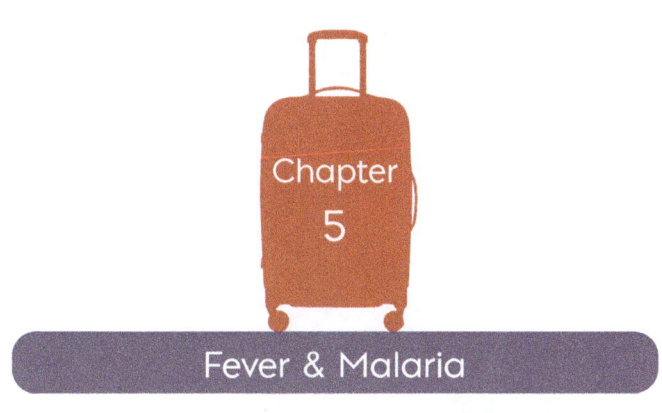

Chapter 5

Fever & Malaria

Fever can be present in many illnesses from cold/virus to Rickettsia/Rocky Mountain Spotted Fever or Lyme disease. Travel to countries within the equator belt are known for viruses carried by mosquitoes such as malaria, yellow fever, Dengue fever, Chikungunya, and Zika. The equator belt is between the Tropic of Cancer and the Tropic of Capricorn lines. A fever (100.4 degrees F or 38 degrees C) is a warning sign for an infectious disease. A fever with an unknown cause after travel to certain countries is suggestive of malaria.

Malaria diagnosed in the USA occurs in people who have traveled to countries known for malaria transmission. Malaria transmitted by a mosquito occurs highly during the rainy seasons (March-May, October-November).

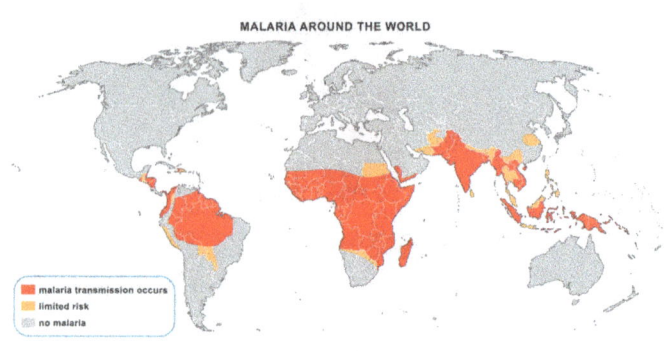

Figure 1. Malaria Around the World Map

Malaria symptoms may show up one to four weeks after the mosquito bite, or it can go undetected for up to one year after being infected. Malaria presents as high fevers, chills, rigors, severe headache; it's cyclic because you will get sick, get better, and then two weeks later you are sick again. The common presentation is shivering and chills for one to two hours, then high fever and sweating followed by a normal temperature. Other symptoms may include fatigue, weakness, nausea, vomiting, diarrhea, dizziness, confusion, disorientation, back pain, and muscle aches. There is a large medication resistance to malaria in some countries; the specific country you traveled to is needed for adequate treatment. Malaria is diagnosed from its presence in your red blood cells. So, you will need medical care as an outpatient or in the hospital depending on the severity of your symptoms.

You can use insect repellent containing 25 percent DEET (adults only) for mosquito bite prevention; repellent with picaridin can be used on children, and natural substances such as lemon eucalyptus oil are recommended. Another preventive measure used to avoid mosquito bites is to keep your skin covered, particularly during dusk and dawn, when mosquitoes are more active. There are prophylactic preventive antimalarial medications available from medical providers; you should take it prior to leaving, during, and after the trip.

Water Accidents & Illnesses

DROWNING

Drowning is the fifth leading cause of unintentional injury in the world. Drowning occurs when a person is submersed under water for a period of time and experiences respiratory impairment. Recognizing someone in distress is crucial to rescue and treatment. If a person is struggling to stay afloat, they may ingest water; and aspiration of the water in the lungs hinders breathing and causes more anxiety and struggling. If you see someone drowning, get a lifeguard and rescue aid immediately. Never try to rescue someone if it puts your life in danger or exceeds your swimming abilities.

Never swim alone and swim with a lifeguard on duty.

DIVE-RELATED ILLNESSES

Diving-related illnesses are related to pressure changes and oxygen/nitrogen gases in our bodies. The air spaces in the body at risk for injury are sinuses, middle ears, intestines, teeth cavities, and lungs.

Some of the diving problems occur suddenly upon surfacing from a dive while others will occur gradually hours to days later. Anyone who has taken diving instruction and received certification is given the signs to look for regarding diving illnesses.

1. The change of barometric pressure with diving squeezes spaces, causing ruptured ear drums (most common and no treatment needed) to lung collapse with difficulty breathing (immediate medical treatment needed).

2. "The Bends" occur when the diver ascends (comes up out of a dive) too fast; nitrogen in the body will form bubbles and disrupt the body tissues. The symptoms vary from fatigue, achy joints, skin rash to difficulty breathing, seizures, paralysis, coma, and

other life-threatening conditions. If you think this has occurred after a dive, go to the nearest hospital as soon as possible.

3. Immediately after ascent of a dive, air bubbles can form in the blood vessels which will result in vertigo (dizziness and spinning), confusion, deafness, blindness, paralysis, or coma. This is life-threatening and should be treated immediately at the nearest hospital.

4. Nitrogen narcosis will occur when a dive is greater than 70 feet (21 meters) below sea level. The nitrogen gas dissolves and affects the brain like alcohol. It occurs suddenly, and the diver becomes confused and disoriented (a clear reason not to dive alone). The treatment is for the diver to ascend to above 65 feet (20 meters) for immediate resolution.

MARINE ANIMAL STINGS

Marine animal stings occur from sea anemones and jellyfish. They can cause intense pain at the site, raised redness, and itching. Occasionally, it will cause nausea and vomiting, pins and needles sensation, and cramps. Jellyfish stings should be washed with vinegar or salt water for thirty minutes as soon as possible to deactivate the venom. You can immerse the area in hot water for twenty minutes to reduce the pain; be careful that the water is not too hot to prevent burning yourself. If tentacles or nematocysts are embedded in the skin, use gloves to carefully remove them with forceps (razor blades or credit cards if forceps are not available). Do not rub with a towel, sand, or use fresh water. It will worsen the condition.

Stingray spines are filled with venom and can puncture the skin. You will experience immediate intense pain. Immerse the area with hot water for thirty to ninety minutes to deactivate the venom. Severe reactions such as difficulty breathing, heart palpitations, weakness, or loss of consciousness require immediate medical treatment.

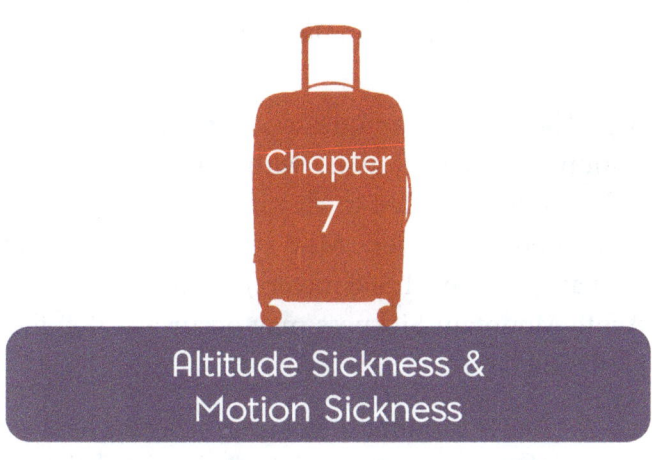

Altitude Sickness & Motion Sickness

Altitude sickness may occur when you ascend 8,000 feet (2,400 meters) above your normal altitude level. This may occur not only when you are hiking the Himalayas or trekking Machu Picchu; it can occur by simply traveling from Florida to Colorado. Altitude sickness is a result of hypoxia (lack of oxygen) at extreme heights. Barometric pressure decreases and causes the red blood cells to carry less oxygen to your organs, mostly the heart and brain. It results in symptoms ranging from mild discomfort to breathing problems and life-threatening conditions.

If you are traveling to an area more than 5,000 feet above your normal altitude and if you plan activity and/or have chronic medical problems, you should consult with your physician prior to the trip. There are techniques and prescription medications to prevent, assist with, and treat altitude sickness. It is divided in classifications of severity: mild, moderate, severe. Mild symptoms can start at least at 5,000 feet (1,500 meters) above sea level and Acute Mountain Sickness may occur at 8,000 feet (2,400 meters).

A. Acute Mountain Sickness – headache, loss of appetite, nausea, insomnia, visual changes or night blindness, weariness, or exhaustion. It has been described as a hangover or flu-like symptoms. If these symptoms occur, stop going higher and use oxygen; spend time at the altitude to become acclimated to height before going higher. If the sickness continues or gets worse, descend.

B. High Altitude Pulmonary Edema – fluid collects in the lungs, dry cough, shortness of breath, chest pain, then cough turns into frothy sputum. If these symptoms occur, descend as soon as possible at least 1,000 to 1,500 feet and use oxygen; a hyperbaric chamber may be needed if symptoms do not improve.

C. High Altitude Cerebral Edema – fluid collecting in the brain, if "B" above is not resolved, which causes increased pressure and affects normal function, loss of coordination, unsteady walking, severe persistent headache, odd behavior, sleepiness, lethargy, unresponsiveness to coma. Medical treatment is needed as soon as possible. Descend and use oxygen, and a hyperbaric chamber may be needed.

- Cusco, Peru: 11,152 feet
- Glacier Peak: 10,542 feet
- Himalayas: 29,029 feet
- Mount Kilimanjaro: 19,341 feet
- Mount Olympus: 9,573 feet
- Mount Rainier: 14,409 feet
- Mount St Helens: 8,366 feet
- Quito, Ecuador: 9,350 feet

Prevention of altitude sickness may reduce the symptoms and severity:

1. Plan your ascent – stop at various altitudes to acclimate (adjust to the new environment),

allowing your body to adjust to the change of atmospheric pressure and oxygen levels; initial acclimation should last for twelve to twenty-four hours after arrival. Professional trekkers will only increase 1,000 to 1,500 feet per night.

2. Avoid intense exercise, which will cause shortness of breath and fatigue.
3. Eat a high carbohydrate diet – 70 percent of the meal should be carbs. Start one to two days prior to ascending to the higher altitude.
4. Stay well-hydrated.
5. Medications prescribed by a physician for altitude sickness can include acetazolamide, nifedipine, or dexamethasone.
6. In Peru, use coca leaves to chew or make tea; it helps with altitude sickness, appetite suppression, and acts as a stimulant to produce energy. When chewing, your cheeks may become numb, but it is not addictive.

MOTION SICKNESS

This condition occurs when your visual movement does not agree with the senses in your brain. You become dizzy, nauseated, and off-balanced, and sometimes, you will vomit. Motion sickness can occur with any form of travel.

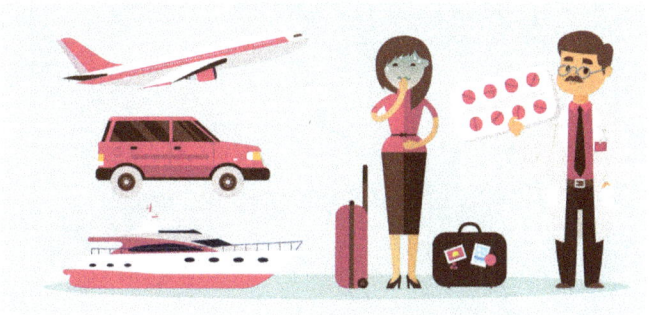

Figure 2. Motion Sickness

In a car, sit in the front seat and focus on the horizon. On an airplane, sit over the wings. On a boat, sit at the center. Aromatherapy oils such as mint and lavender are helpful as are ginger candies to calm the nausea.

If you are prone to having severe motion sickness or have had it before, contact your doctor for medication. If you plan to be on a boat for more than three days, patches are available for a steady infusion of medications. Keep in mind that some of these medications have side effects such as sleepiness and drowsiness.

Chapter 8

Environmental Problems

Environmental medical emergencies related to heat or cold occur while travelers venture into another environment, whether hiking, trekking, biking, or running. Often, the emergency will occur in remote areas where immediate medical assistance is not available. Basic prevention such as wearing protective clothing, wearing layers, and limiting exposure time can save limbs and lives.

HEAT-RELATED ILLNESSES

It occurs when the body temperature regulation is disrupted and the body overheats. It can occur due to overexposure to the environment and during vigorous physical activity. Prevent heat-related illnesses by avoiding long hours of exposure in the heat or direct sunlight; avoid direct sunlight during the hottest hours of 10 a.m. to 4 p.m. Be careful while vacationing within the equator sunbelt region if you are not used to the harsh sun.

HEAT CRAMPS

Heat cramps are uncontrolled muscle spasms that can occur while the body is overheating. It is due to dehydration and depletion of salt in the body. The spasms occur suddenly and are painful. Stretching the muscle and direct pressure on the spasm will slowly provide resolution. Hydration and salt/electrolyte replacement is advised.

HEAT EXHAUSTION

Heat exhaustion occurs when the body temperature rises accompanied by dehydration. Heat exhaustion is serious but reversible with quick treatment. Symptoms include excessive sweating, pale skin, nausea and vomiting, headache, and weakness. Treatment includes stopping the activity, taking the person to a cool/shaded environment, loosening tight restrictive clothing, lying down with feet elevated if dizzy, spraying misty water on the person, applying a cool wet cloth to the face, neck, and chest, placing ice in the armpits, using a fan for cooling, and drinking fluids. If no improvement occurs, seek medical treatment.

HEAT STROKE

Heat stroke is considered a medical emergency. The body temperature rises, the temperature regulation center malfunctions or is overwhelmed, and the body's cooling mechanisms (sweating and evaporation) are no longer working. The symptoms include body hot to touch, dry, red skin, nausea and vomiting, confusion, dizziness, and sometimes unconscious or seizures. Call EMS for immediate medical treatment. While waiting, cool down the person. Move them to a cool and shaded environment; pour cold water on the body or place ice/cold packs around neck, armpits, and groin. Also, use a fan to enhance cooling.

COLD-RELATED ILLNESSES

Cool or cold environments along with wetness can cause severe, decreased inner core body temperature.

HYPOTHERMIA

Hypothermia is one of the most dangerous cold temperature emergencies. This occurs when your body temperature is lower than the set point in the brain and your normal body function. Hypothermia shows up in different stages: mild, moderate, and severe. Hypothermia occurs when there is extended exposure to a cold environment, so prevention is the key point.

- Proper clothing protects the body from hypothermia. Sounds simple, right? You should know the temperature of your travel destination and take the appropriate clothes. In a cold environment, choose materials that will maintain your body heat even if it should get wet. Consider waterproof clothing if activities will cause you to get wet.

- Layering of clothes will maintain body heat, and allow you to cool off by removing a layer if needed and adding a layer if you become cold. Consider a base layer of synthetic material which allows moisture to wick away from the body.

- Watch for signs of hypothermia and never travel alone in a severe cold environment.

How do you know if you are cold and going toward hypothermia? The first symptom is shivering.

Mild symptoms – skin is pale, cold to touch, shivering, loss of fine coordination of movement, normal mental status. Treat this by warming the body, removing wet clothing if necessary, covering the head and neck (areas of most heat loss); a warm, sweet, nonalcoholic drink will provide warmth and heat generating carbohydrates. Apply hot packs or hot water bottles to the torso or move the body to increase internal heat production.

Moderate symptoms – The person has controlled shivering, confusion, sluggish movements, slurred speech, poor coordination, and altered gait. These can be called "fumbling, grumbling, mumbling, and stumbling." Immediate treatment is necessary. Place the person in a warm environment; actively rewarm the person with heat (hot packs, hot water bottles, warm towels) on the torso, armpits, and back; provide a warm, sweet, nonalcoholic liquid; wrap the person with warm clothing/blanket to trap internal heat; avoid excessive movement.

Severe symptoms – Shivering will stop; the person gets muscle stiffness, confusion to coma, decrease of heart rate and breathing. IMMEDIATE medical treatment is needed. Prevent persistent heat loss and move the person to a warm environment if possible; protect them from the environment. Be gentle and careful with the person because severe cold can cause irregular heartbeats. Do not give anything to eat or drink to avoid aspiration in the lungs. Wrap the person in an insulation wrap (inner insulation layer with outer waterproof layer to trap heat next to the body).

FROSTBITE

Frostbite occurs when the skin freezes, and the tissue underneath is damaged. It normally occurs in fingers, toes, or the end of a limb. The skin turns red to white and pale; the skin becomes firm and hard. There is numbness, loss of sensation, and pain in the frostbite area. Take the person to a warm environment and remove any wet clothing from the skin. Do not rub or massage the area. For treatment, submerge the area in warm (not hot) water. Wrap the area with clean cloth/towel as if it were a burn; place pads between the fingers or toes, so they don't stick together.

To prevent frostbite:

- Limit your time in the cold
- Dress in layers of clothes
- Protect your fingers/toes with waterproof, insulated gloves/socks; moisture wicking
- Cover your head and ears/protect from wind
- Shoes or boots should fit properly, not too tight to restrict blood flow
- Treat mild frostbite immediately and re-warm area
- Do not touch cold metal with bare hands

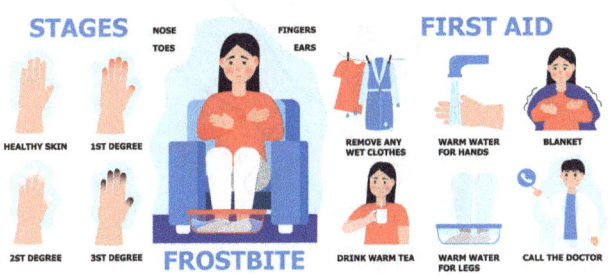

Figure 3. Stages of Frost Bite & Treatment

SUN BLINDNESS (PHOTOKERATITIS)

The sun shining off of snow, water, ice, or sand can damage the eye with UV ray exposure. Symptoms include eye pain, redness, swelling, blurry vision, sensitivity to light, gritty feeling in eyes, headache, seeing halos, twitching eyelids, or temporary loss of vision. Remove contact lenses if wearing, apply cold cloth over eyes, and avoid rubbing your eyes. The symptoms usually resolve within twenty-four to forty-eight hours. To prevent photokeratitis, wear sunglasses or goggles with UVA/UVB protection.

SNAKE BITES

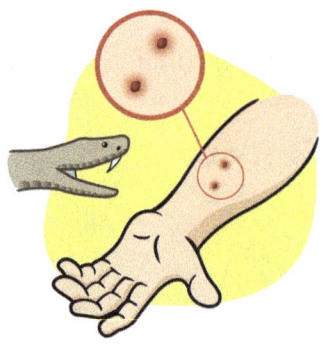

Figure 4. Snake Bite

There are venomous (poisonous) and nonvenomous snakes. The saying "Red on yellow kills a fellow. Red on black, venom lack" helps to identify venomous versus nonvenomous coral snakes by their color pattern. Coral snakes bite, chew, and fix their fangs into the bite. There is pain and swelling at the bite site, but other symptoms will lag in time including abdominal pain, nausea and vomiting, increased and racing heart rate, difficulty breathing, drooling, and change of mental status. Pit viper snakes are cottonmouths, copperheads, and rattlesnakes. They strike quickly and only once, leaving a single or double fang bite. There will be intense pain, burning, and rapid swelling.

If bitten, immediate medical care is necessary. On the way, wrap a snug but not too tight bandage around the bite, and keep the area below the heart. DO NOT cool the area, use a tourniquet on the limb, cut the wound, or try to suck out the venom.

TICK BITES

Ticks are insects found in tall grass, shrubs, and bushes; travelers experience ticks adhering to their skin while hiking and trekking through the woods and fields. Ticks will transmit diseases such as

Lyme Disease or Rocky Mountain Spotted Fever. If you notice a tick on your skin, remove it completely with tweezers, pulling straight off with a steady, slow motion. Clean the area with soap and water. If part of the tick remains, you may develop a rash, fever, or flu-like symptoms. Seek medical treatment for removal of the remaining segment.

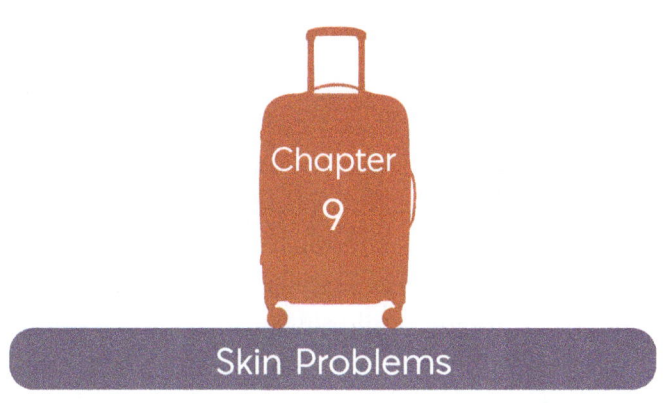

Chapter 9

Skin Problems

BUG BITES

Many diseases and parasites are carried by mosquitoes, ticks, fleas, and flies. Here is a very short list of what some bugs carry:

- Mosquitoes: dengue, chikungunya, malaria, Zika, yellow fever, Japanese encephalitis.
- Ticks: African tick-bite fever, Mediterranean spotted fever, tick-borne encephalitis.
- Others: scrub typhus (chiggers), plague (fleas), sleeping sickness (tsetse flies).

As mentioned earlier, you may need pre-travel medications as disease prevention from these bites. They can be prescribed by your primary care physician, a walk-in clinic, a travel clinic, or telemedicine visits.

When traveling to an area that is known to have one or many of these diseases, wear insect repellent (natural-oil of lemon eucalyptus or chemical), particularly during the dusk and dawn periods. Adults can use an insect repellent that has DEET 25 percent or greater; children should not use DEET, but instead use repellent with Picaridin or natural repellent products. In addition, wear long sleeves and pants in areas where you might be exposed to insects. At night, sleep in a screened area with a net over your bed or sleeping bag. Unusual bug bites can also infect you with parasites.

If you develop a fever after a bite and the wound does not heal or you experience generalized illness, see a physician as soon as possible. If you have returned to the US, inform your medical provider of the country to which you traveled. Malaria may not show up for one year after infection.

Stings from bees, wasps, or fire ants will cause pain at the bite site, redness, swelling, and itching. If the stinger of the bee is in the skin, remove it as soon as possible. Wash the stung area with soap and water, use cooling or anti-itch ointment for pain and swelling, and cover the area.

SUNBURNS

A sunburn is considered a first-degree burn (extreme redness and pain) or second-degree burn (redness, pain, and blisters). While you should always use sunscreen as protection, you must also limit your time of exposure to UV rays. Water, snow, and sand can intensify the sun rays, which means that the beach is not the only place you get sun exposure; it can happen while hiking, skiing, mountain climbing, or being anywhere within the equator belt. While in the equator belt (between the Tropic of Cancer and Tropic of Capricorn), you can burn within twenty minutes of exposure since you are closest to the sun. In general, avoid direct exposure between 10:00 am to 4:00 pm.

Sunscreen should be applied at least twenty minutes prior to the exposure; this is how long it takes for it to be absorbed into the skin cells. Use a broad-spectrum UVA/UVB sunscreen with 30 SPF or higher. Reapply every two hours or after you've been in the water. Remember to put it on the top of your head, face, ears, and back of the neck. Lips should also be protected with a lip balm, SPF 15 or greater.

To treat a sunburn, stay out of the sun for a few days (forty-eight hours for second-degree burns), apply cool compresses on the affected area, take cold showers, get lots of fluids, take pain relievers if necessary, and apply aloe to keep the burned skin moisturized. If you must go in the sun, cover the sunburned skin properly. If a large surface area of your body is sunburned, you can develop sun toxicity or poisoning. Along with the blistering skin, you will experience swelling, tingling, headache, fever, nausea, dehydration, and dizziness. If this occurs, seek medical treatment as soon as possible.

BLISTERS

Blisters are common with hikers or first-time walking tourists. Blisters form from friction and heat, shoes too tight or too loose, or walking in new shoes that are not broken in or that conform to your foot. Treatment of a blister is with a blister pad or moleskin.

SKIN INFECTIONS

Insect bites can present symptoms such as minor itching and redness to hot, inflamed, and infected skin. If you get bitten, try not to scratch the area. I know that's a hard task. Your fingers and nails may carry microscopic dirt, and when scratched, the bacteria may enter beneath the skin. Also, your skin has natural bacteria living on the outside but will cause an infection once they enter underneath the skin. MRSA, a penicillin resistant bacterium, is one example. For itchy bites, use calamine or Benadryl ointment directly on the area. Minor cuts on your skin also get infected from an unpurified water source. So, shaving with the water in undeveloped countries or swimming in lakes with open wounds can produce skin infections. Neosporin ointment can be used on minor skin infections and keep the area clean and dry. Dog bites, cat bites, or cat scratches can fester into a skin infection called cellulitis. Once again, keep the wound clean and dry and use an antibacterial ointment directly on the wound.

If you notice an area that has become red, warm to the touch, painful, and/or draining yellow fluid, you want to seek medical attention. If you see red streaks going away from the infection toward the upper body, you may need intravenous antibiotics to avoid spreading the infection within your body.

PLANTAR WARTS/FEET FUNGUS

Your feet are an entry point into your body, similar to your mouth. As you walk along the rocky beaches of the world, cutting the soles of your feet or standing in the shower of your hotel in an underdeveloped country, remember to protect your feet. The bottom surface of your feet is called the "plantar" region. Bacteria, viruses, and parasites (worms) can enter the plantar surface of the feet when defects are present. These organisms enter the body and travel within the blood, while others only affect the surface skin like plantar warts.

Plantar warts are caused by a virus (human papillomavirus) and enter the plantar surface through minor cuts and scrapes. It's highly contagious and may spread on surfaces, like pools, showers, or gym surfaces. Warts may not appear until weeks after initial exposure. Most adults have built up an immunity to the virus, and it is seen more commonly in children. However, adults with weakened immune systems are at risk of getting plantar warts.

Plantar warts only remain on the surface of the skin and are somewhat "harmless." The major complaint is the pain they cause. Calluses form to prevent the spread of warts, but pressure and constant walking on the feet cause pain. The typical wart will go away without any treatment. They appear as small bumps on the soles of the feet (possible dark dots on the surface) and cause pain in the area when standing or walking. If the area becomes red, hot to the touch, and more tender, an infection may have developed. You need to seek medical treatment.

An item I always include in my international pack is duct tape. Duct tape? How is that connected to plantar warts? Warts will soften when duct tape is placed over them for a prolonged period and will reduce your pain. DO NOT attempt to cut them off – you may cause more harm. Other treatments used are topical solutions (salicylic acid), burning, or freezing, but the best way is prevention.

Another foot problem is fungus, or tinea pedis. You can catch the fungus through direct contact with an infected person, or by touching surfaces contaminated with the fungus. The fungus thrives in warm, moist environments such as showers, on locker room floors, and around swimming pools.

Situations that cause feet fungal infections include:

- visiting public places barefoot, especially locker rooms, showers, and swimming pools

- sharing socks, shoes, or towels with an infected person
- wearing tight, closed-toe shoes
- keeping your feet wet for long periods of time
- having sweaty feet
- having a minor skin or nail injury on your foot

Symptoms of a fungal infection are itching, stinging, and burning between your toes or on the soles of your feet; blisters on your feet that itch; cracking and peeling skin on your feet, most commonly between your toes and on your soles; raw skin on your feet; discolored, thick, and crumbly toenails; or toenails that pull away from the nail bed. If you have any of these symptoms, seek medical help. It can be treated with anti-fungal ointment (over-the-counter or prescribed) and/or oral medications. Home remedies include soaking your feet in salt water or vinegar water to dry up the blisters. And tea tree oil has shown to progress healing. Keep your feet dry, wear breathable shoes and socks, use anti-fungal powder, and don't share socks and shoes.

The ultimate treatment of summer feet infections is PREVENTION. So, purchase those roll up shower shoes or dollar store flip-flops for the pools and showers. It will only add three to four ounces to your bag. You can also place them in the outside pocket of your carry-on. If you don't have the shoes, remember to wash your feet with disinfectant soap after walking barefoot on those surfaces. Also, keep the soles and heels moisturized to avoid dry skin cracks.

CONTACT DERMATITIS

This is an allergic reaction of the skin when it comes in "contact" with an irritant. It presents as dry, scaly skin, redness, blisters, hives, darkened skin, itching, burning, swelling, and sensitivity. It may have the shape of the object of contact (metal against skin) or where the skin was touched (poison ivy). Common products that cause contact dermatitis are jewelry (metal with nickel or gold), latex, chemicals, poison ivy or oak, and skin care products. Avoid scratching the irritated area and clean with warm, soapy water to remove the irritant. Stop using any of the skin products and wash all clothes with possible poison ivy/oak oils on them. If the rash is close to the eyes, mouth, or a large part of the body, seek medical treatment.

Most skin rashes and problems can be treated with topical corticosteroids, oral antihistamines, pain reliever medication, and antibiotic ointment if needed.

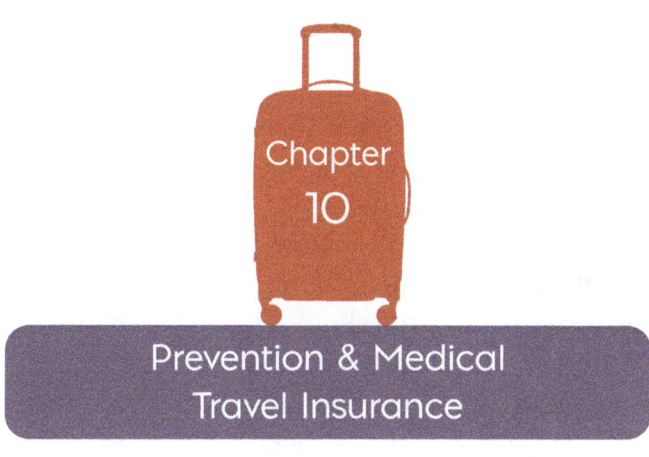

Chapter 10

Prevention & Medical Travel Insurance

You book your honeymoon, second honeymoon, trip of a lifetime, or a luxury getaway. It's ten months away, and you have a steady payment plan. The tours are organized, your trip is paid for, you are ready, and your excitement builds, and then life happens.

Travel insurance is an expense that should always be added into the budget. You can buy insurance when you purchase airline tickets and/or book a vacation package. If you are a business traveler or go on more than two international trips per year, you should consider an annual travel insurance policy. It can be bought through the airlines, your credit card company, your travel agent, or independent travel insurance agencies. Policies vary and can compensate for events such as delay of travel (you missed a flight and then missed the cruise), delay of bags (greater than six hours), loss of bags, and even cancellation of a trip for any reason.

Medical travel insurance is a necessity while traveling internationally. If you become ill or have an accident while traveling, your US based medical insurance typically will not cover your medical care internationally, but more importantly, most international medical facilities will not accept it. Medical facilities not in the US will require payment before service in the form of cash or credit card. To be seen in an A&E (emergency room) in a foreign country is not as costly as in the USA, but it can be a nuisance, timely, and disrupt your vacation. Medical travel insurance is helpful because it can be accepted by international medical facilities, or you are reimbursed for your payment upon your return home. You can obtain assistance in finding services nearby for your medical need, and if necessary, you can be evacuated to a higher-level care facility in another country or back to the USA. There are different types of medical travel insurance available: one-time vacation, annual traveler, business traveler, adventurer, student abroad, mission traveler, and more. The cost of medical travel insurance is usually dependent on the cost of the trip and the age of the traveler. Medical travel insurance will add a little extra cost to your vacation, but it saves you a large amount of anxiety, frustration, and money, if medical care is needed.

TRAVELING WITH MEDICATIONS

Pre-travel medications for nausea, motion sickness, diarrhea, malaria, and other travel-related illnesses can be prescribed by your physician, a walk-in clinic, or a travel clinic. There are requirements for traveling internationally with prescribed medications, and some countries restrict certain drugs even if it is medically indicated.

Medications in foreign countries may be different, have a different name, come in different packing, and/or be written in an unknown language. It is best for you to travel with your prescribed medications and your favorite over-the-counter medications because you may not find them in the country of your destination. Your prescription medications should be in the original bottles with your name on the bottle and packed in the carry-on bag. Do not mix different types of pills in one bottle. If you are stopped by customs, your bottles may be inspected to verify the medication matches the label on the bottle.

Entering another country with unmarked medication can be considered drug trafficking, as returning to the USA with various unknown medications will be flagged as drug trafficking. The medications can be confiscated and destroyed, and you may be detained or even jailed. If you are carrying narcotics, sleep aids, anxiety medications, or injectable medications, you should have a note from the prescribing physician on letterhead paper. Be aware that some countries do not allow you to bring controlled substances even if they have been prescribed.

MEDICAL TREATMENT IN A FOREIGN COUNTRY

Medical care in other countries may vary in quality and accessibility. You can check with the hotel concierge for a suitable medical facility, one that has English-speaking doctors. As mentioned previously, you will likely be expected to pay for your care with cash or a credit card. The US Embassy or consulate can help in obtaining the appropriate medical care while traveling and assist in evacuation if needed. If the US government evacuates you due to medical reasons, you are still required to pay for the services.

If you have a chronic illness or are going on an adventurous trip, research of medical facilities and locations should be done in advance of your travel. Two resources to use are International Society of Travel Medicine (www.istm.org) or International Association of Medical Assistance to Travelers (www.iamat.org). Plan by seeing your primary care physician before your trip for possible vaccinations or prophylactic medications for illnesses.

Chapter 11

First Aid as a Non-Medical Traveler–Accidents, Cuts, and Recognizing a Medical Emergency

Have you ever had a cut and couldn't get help right away? Twisted an ankle while hiking and there's no cell phone service? Wondered if a problem is a true emergency? This chapter will address some basic first aid techniques to know while traveling if immediate medical help is not available.

BURNS

A burn is caused by direct skin contact with flames, hot objects or liquids, electricity, or chemicals.

Minor burns can be taken care of with cool water, keeping the wound clean and dry, and pain relief medications.

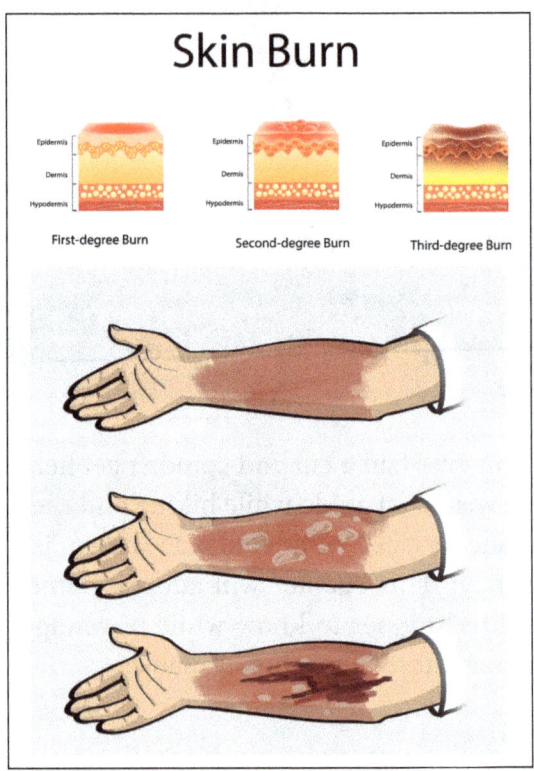

Figure 5. Burns

Severe burns involve depth of the skin, blisters, skin peeling, and large areas of burned skin. Burns of the face, neck, hands, feet, or genitals need medical treatment.

If a fire happens, stop, drop, and roll. Smother the fire with cloth and splash with water, except if the fire is caused by oil/grease. Remove any clothing that was burning off the person to prevent continuous injury. Remove any metal jewelry from the burned area. DO NOT USE butter, honey, or potato peels.

All electrical burns caused by DC/AC current or lightning strikes need medical treatment.

CHEMICALS IN THE EYE

If chemicals splash in the eye, flush the eye immediately with large amounts of water. Open the eye and flush continuously for approximately fifteen minutes. Seek immediate medical treatment.

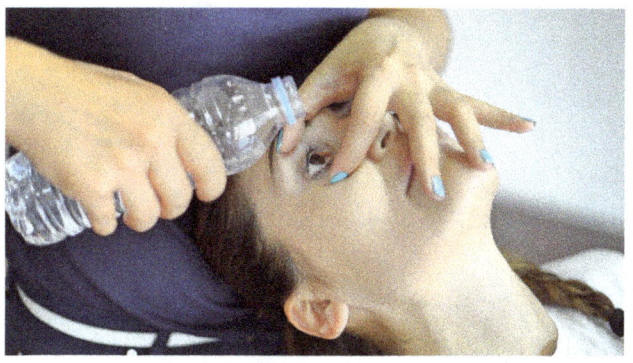

Figure 6. Eye Wash

CONTROL OF BLEEDING

Find the area on the body that is bleeding, expose it, and with a clean pad or cloth, apply direct pressure on the site. Direct pressure on a wound works well and is the first treatment method to treat a bleeding wound. If you have rolled gauze, you can wrap the gauze around it to hold the pressure. If the blood soaks through, leave it in place and use another pad or cloth, pressing down firmly. Do not use a tourniquet or tie off an arm or leg without training.

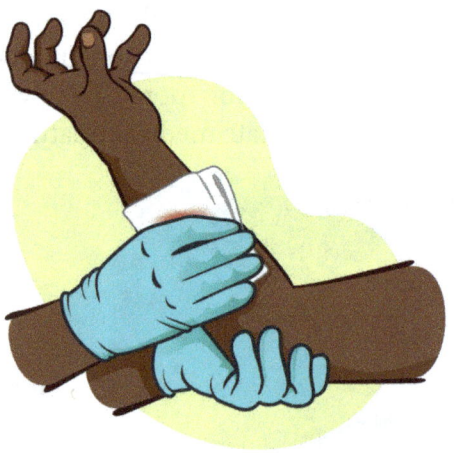

Figure 7. Compression to Control Bleeding

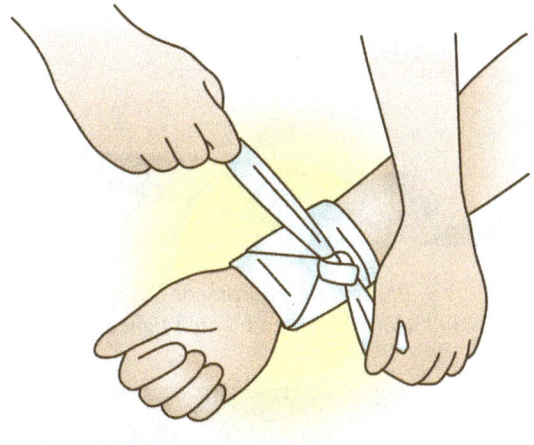

Figure 8. Compression Bandaging

FAINTING

Fainting is a temporary loss of consciousness, but the cause may not be known. If no injury is apparent, lay the person flat and raise their feet with an object underneath, then call EMS. Loosen any restrictive clothing like ties, scarves, and belts. If the person hits their head while fainting, lay them flat, stabilize the head by putting something on each side of the head, and do not move them. Call EMS immediately.

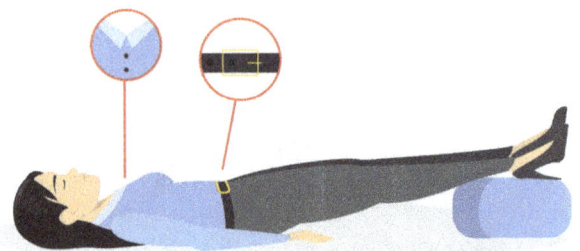

Figure 9. Position for Fainting or Dizzy Persons (lay flat, elevate legs, and loosen tight clothing)

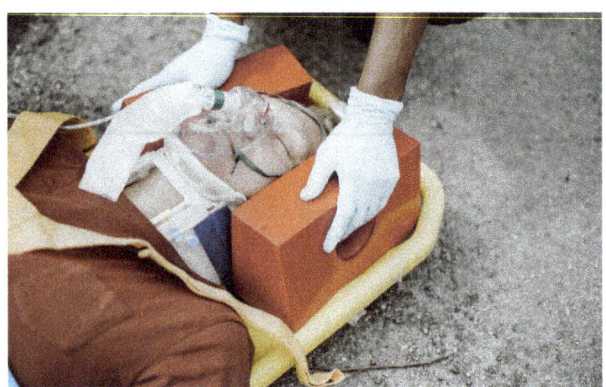

Figure 10. Stabilize the Head and Neck with Injury

LIMB INJURY – ARM OR LEG

You stepped off the curb and twisted your ankle; you fell onto your hand and your wrist aches. You twisted your knee while hiking and cannot put weight on the leg; you are out of cellular range. What do you do? Of course, you packed one or two ace wrap bandages. These wraps are stretchy and provide compression on a joint, muscle, or bone to stabilize the injury, sprain, or fracture. If you need more reinforcement, make a splint. Use a solid, firm object (board, tree limbs, books, or magazine for example) on each side of the joint injured, and then wrap it to make the joint/bone immobile.

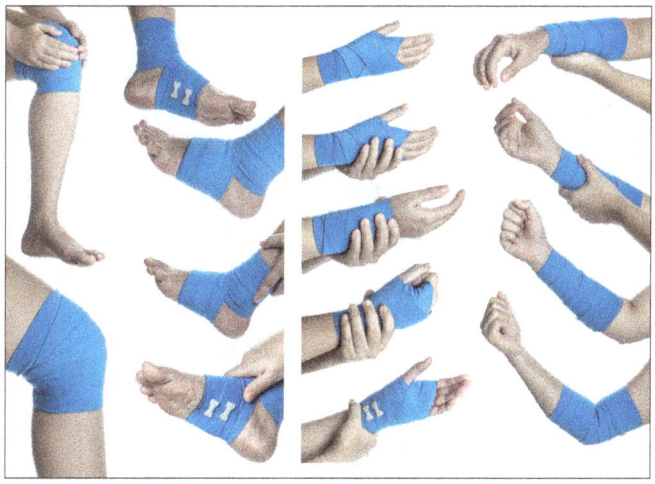

Figures 11 and 12. Ace Wrap to a Joint

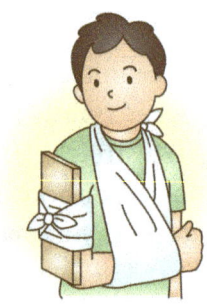 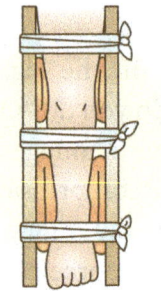

Figures 13 and 14. Make a Splint to Stabilize a Broken Bone

PUNCTURE WOUNDS

If an object impales or penetrates the body, do not pull it out. Prevent movement of the body part in order to prevent further injury. If you can, wrap it at the base of the object/skin connection, and transport the person for medical treatment. An object in the eye requires seeking medical treatment immediately.

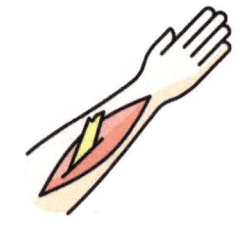

Figure 15. Puncture Wound

RECOGNIZING MEDICAL EMERGENCIES

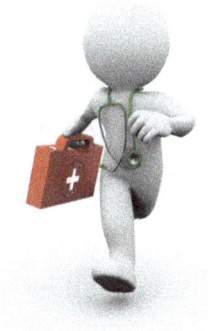

Figure 16. Medical Emergencies

In the USA, 911 is the number to call for Emergency Medical Services and an ambulance. It is not the same in countries outside of the USA. Know the emergency call number of your destination or how to seek immediate emergency medical care. At hotels, you can call the concierge desk for medical help.

Medical emergencies are just that, an emergency; an unexpected event due to medical conditions or illnesses. You should suspect a medical emergency if the person suddenly becomes weak, confused, has severe pain, trouble breathing, or becomes unconscious without warning.

ALLERGIC REACTIONS OR ANAPHYLAXIS

An allergic reaction is exposure to a previous allergen that causes an overabundant histamine response when re-exposed. The cause of the allergy is usually food, medications, and stings. The person will develop hives, swelling of the lips and tongue, itchy throat, difficulty breathing/wheezing, and hypotension (low blood pressure). THIS IS A MEDICAL EMERGENCY and LIFE-THREATENING. Immediate medical attention is needed to prevent the airway from closing up and breathing being affected. People who have known allergies (nuts, bees, etc.) may carry medication called an EpiPen. This medicine is an auto-injection of epinephrine into the body to slow down the allergic reaction. If the person is unable to give it to themselves, press the opening of the injector pen to the leg or arm (even through clothing) and follow the directions. Anyone that needs to use an EpiPen must be taken to the nearest hospital for further care because the medication is only effective for a limited amount of time.

ALTERED MENTAL STATUS

Many medical conditions can cause a person to suddenly not act normal, undergo personality or behavior changes, or become unconscious.

- Call EMS for immediate medical treatment.
- Keep the person calm and comfortable – in the position they choose.
- If unconscious, lay them flat and roll them to their left side if they have not had an injury.

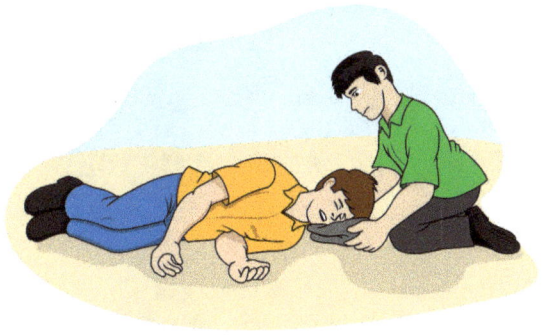

Figure 17. Stabilize a Sick Person

SHOCK

Shock occurs when the person has low blood flow to the body tissues. Severe dehydration or continuous loss of blood can put someone into shock. If the person is irritable, restless, pale, confused, and their skin is cool and clammy, call emergency services and get them medical help immediately. While waiting for help: 1) lay the person flat 2) maintain body temperature, you may need to cover them up 3) place something under their feet to elevate their legs and 4) keep them comfortable and calm.

Chapter 12

Post-Travel Illnesses

If you get sick after your travels, please see a medical provider as soon as possible. Let them know you were recently traveling, where you traveled and if anything occurred like injury, insect bite, foods eaten, body fluid exposures, medical procedures (Medical Tourism), tattoos or piercings. We can alter the physical examination and tests accordingly to diseases not usually occurring or search for unusual sources of the illness.

The most common conditions that travelers experience when returning home are:

- Upset stomach/diarrhea
- Fever
- Skin and soft tissue issues
- Breathing problems
- Malaise

The questions your medical professional will want to know answers to are:

- Where have you traveled in the last six to eight weeks? USA or internationally?
- How long were you traveling? Where did you stay (hotel, private home, tent)?
- What was your last meal before you became sick? Cooked at home, dining out, street food, drinks, etc.?
- When did your symptoms initiate? Before, during, or after your travels?
- Is anyone else who traveled with you ill?
- What did you do on your trip?
- Were you bitten by bugs or animals? Exposed to animals?
- Did you swim in fresh water?
- Did you receive health care abroad?
- Any other possible exposures (sex, tattoos, piercings)?

DIARRHEA

We talked about traveler's diarrhea before. However, if you have persistent diarrhea (ten or more stools in a day or diarrhea lasting more than two days), we want to discover the source and treat accordingly.

Common bacteria that cause diarrhea are E. coli (different types), giardia, shigella, or vibrio. Each bacterium presents differently, so doctors will want to know about your stool. What color is it? Does it have a smell? Is there blood, mucous, or a greasy appearance? Is it loose, runny, or watery? Do you have abdominal cramping, gas, or bloating? Most likely, you'll be asked to provide a stool sample for testing. Your doctor will then prescribe you the right medication to treat the bacteria, or in some cases, worms and parasites from water sources that also cause diarrhea.

FEVER

A fever is a common symptom in many illnesses. However, a fever is most concerning when you have been traveling in the equator belt (between Tropic of Cancer and Tropic of Capricorn). Countries within the belt are known for viruses carried by mosquitoes: malaria, yellow fever, Dengue fever, chikungunya, and Zika. Malaria, for instance, manifests as high fevers, chills, rigors, and severe headache; plus, it's cyclic, meaning you will get sick, get better, and then, two weeks later, get sick again.

Some forms of malaria have a medication resistance, so your doctor will need to know the specific country you visited. Then, they will diagnose you based on whether they find malaria in your red blood cells. Preventive antimalarial medications are available from medical providers, so take it prior to the trip, during the trip, and after the trip.

DEHYDRATION

When dehydrated, you may experience symptoms such as muscle aches, soreness, joint pain, fatigue, and possibly fever. In severe cases, it will lead to rhabdomyolysis. Your muscles break down, and the resulting product (lactic acid) is a large molecule that gets stuck in your kidneys and causes kidney failure. You will require a large amount of fluids intravenously for rehydration and may require hospitalization.

RASH

You may develop a rash from exposure to different plants and vegetation, your clothes being washed in a foreign country's water and detergent, bug bites, and various other scenarios. Inform your medical provider of the country you visited and possible things you came into contact with such as bugs or chemicals. Also, consider insect or bed bug bites from the travel.

RESPIRATORY ILLNESSES

Cough and difficulty breathing presents with a respiratory illness usually due to a virus. There are known international illnesses from certain areas such as SARS, MERS, or Avian Flu. You can also develop lung irritants while participating in activities such as sand dune riding in the desert or spelunking in the bat caves of the southeastern USA. If you have asthma, emphysema, or any lung disease, take precautions while traveling by using a facial mask. If you develop trouble breathing, pneumonia, or severe allergies following your travel, seek medical help. Breathing difficulties can also be a presentation of blood clots.

***

Addendum:
As of March 2020, SARS-CoV2 (COVID-19) was declared a respiratory disease and pandemic by the

World Health Organization. It is advised and mandated in some countries to wear masks/face coverings to prevent transmission of the disease. Social distancing (6 feet or 2 meters) and frequent hand washing are also recommended to reduce the spread of the disease.

Appendix

SEXUAL TRANSMITTED ILLNESSES

No judgment. Information is given only to keep you healthy and safe.

It has been estimated that 20 percent of travelers will have casual sex with an unknown partner. And other avenues of getting a sexually transmitted illness include sex tourism, commercial sex workers, and college spring break. The familiar STIs include gonorrhea, chlamydia, herpes, and HIV. An uncommon but prevalent STI is shigellosis. Shigella is a bacterium that is found in the stool and will cause severe diarrhea; it may still be present up to two weeks after the diarrhea has ceased. MSM may develop shigellosis along with WSM when anal sex is followed by vaginal sex; shigella also have been shown on the skin of the thighs and buttocks.

The best way is prevention and following safe sex practices:

1. Wash your hands, genitals, and anus with soap and water before and after sex.
2. Use a barrier method (condoms) correctly with oral, vaginal, and anal sex to reduce your risk of infection transmission.

3. Wash sex toys with soap and water after each use. Only use water-based lubricant on toys because silicon will break down material and cause cracks holding bacteria.//
4. Don't assume your partner is STI free because of no signs or symptoms. Talk openly about it and find out their last date of testing.
5. Consider getting vaccinated for Hepatitis B.

MEDICAL RESOURCES TO CONSIDER WHILE TRAVELING

1. Urgent care centers
2. Walk-in clinics
3. Telemedicine apps for the phone or tablet with either telephone or video capability.
4. Hotel concierge for recommendations of medical sources and English-speaking doctors

EMERGENCY CONTACT NUMBERS
(not inclusive of all countries)

- Australia: 000 (cell phone: 112)
- Bahamas: 911
- Barbados: 119
- Belgium: 101 (cell phone: 112)
- Bermuda: 911
- Brazil: 911
- Canada: 911
- Columbia: 119
- Croatia: 112
- Denmark: 112
- Dominica Republic: 911
- Finland: 112
- France: 112
- Germany: 112
- Haiti: 118
- Hong Kong: 999
- Jamaica: 110
- Kenya: 999
- South Korea: 119
- Mexico: 065
- Morocco: 15
- New Zealand: 111
- Philippines: 166, 117
- Portugal: 112
- Saudi Arabia: 997
- South Africa: 10177
- South Africa-Cape Town: 107
- Switzerland: 144
- Taiwan: 119
- Thailand: 191
- UAE: 998, 999
- United Kingdom: 999
- Vatican City: 113
- Venezuela: 171
- Vietnam: 05
- Zambia: 999

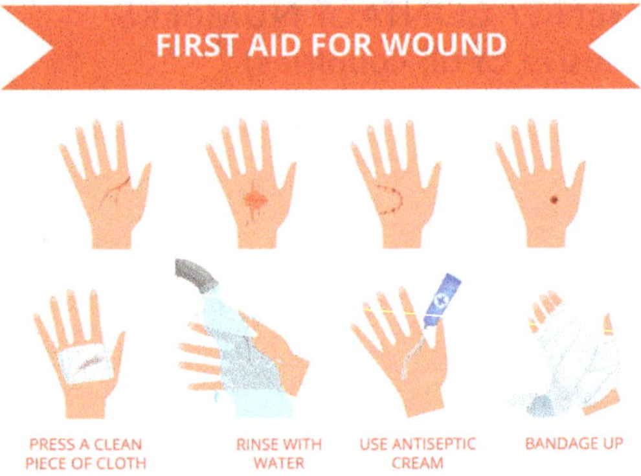

FIRST AID FOR WOUND
PRESS A CLEAN PIECE OF CLOTH
RINSE WITH WATER
USE ANTISEPTIC CREAM
BANDAGE UP

Figure 18. First Aid for Wound

Heimlich Maneuver

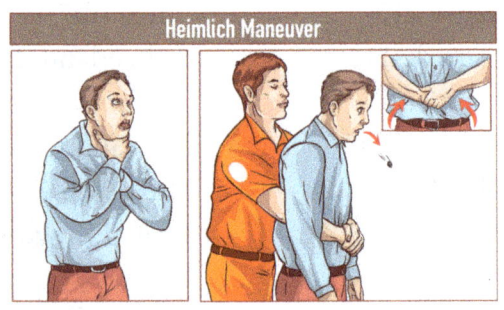

Figure 19. Heimlich Maneuver for Choking

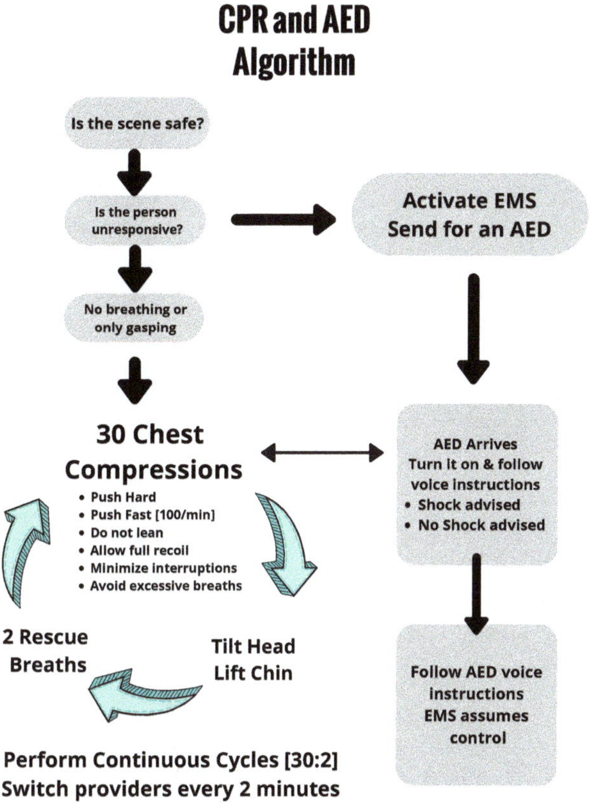

CPR and AED Algorithm

Is the scene safe?

↓

Is the person unresponsive? → **Activate EMS Send for an AED**

↓

No breathing or only gasping

↓

30 Chest Compressions
- Push Hard
- Push Fast [100/min]
- Do not lean
- Allow full recoil
- Minimize interruptions
- Avoid excessive breaths

↔ **AED Arrives Turn it on & follow voice instructions**
- Shock advised
- No Shock advised

↓

Follow AED voice instructions EMS assumes control

2 Rescue Breaths — **Tilt Head Lift Chin**

Perform Continuous Cycles [30:2]
Switch providers every 2 minutes

Figure 20. CPR & AED Algorithm

References

"10 Dangerous Food Safety Mistakes." CDC. https://www.cdc.gov/foodsafety/ten-dangerous-mistakes.html.

"2020 American Heart Association Guidelines for CPR and ECC." CPR & First Aid, Emergency Cardiovascular Care. American Heart Association. https://cpr.heart.org/en/resuscitation-science/cpr-and-ecc-guidelines.

American Safety and Institute. 2018. *ASHI Wilderness First Aid Version 8.0 Instructor Guide.*

Bradley A. Connor. "Travelers' Diarrhea." CDC. https://wwwnc.cdc.gov/travel/yellowbook/aaaaaaaaaaaaaaaa2020/preparing-international-travelers/travelers-diarrhea.

"Food Poisoning Symptoms." CDC. https://www.cdc.gov/foodsafety/symptoms.html.

International Society of Travel Medicine. *Travel Medicine Review and Update Course.* 2018.

"Older Travelers." Travel.State.Gov. https://travel.state.gov/content/travel/en/international-travel/before-you-go/travelers-with-special-considerations/info-older-travelers.html.

R. M. Merchant, A. A. Topjian, A. R. Panchal, A. Cheng, K. Aziz, K. M. Berg, E. J. Lavonas, and D. J. Magid. "Part 1: Executive Summary: 2020 American Heart Association Guidelines for Cardiopulmonary Resuscitation and Emergency Cardiovascular Care." Circulation. 2020;142(suppl 2):S337–S357. doi: 10.1161/CIR.0000000000000918.

R. W. Neumar, M. Shuster, C. W. Callaway, L. M. Gent, D. L. Atkins, F. Bhanji, S. C. Brooks, A. R. de Caen, M. W. Donnino, and J. M. Ferrer, et al. "Part 1: Executive Summary: 2015 American Heart Association Guidelines Update for Cardiopulmonary Resuscitation and Emergency Cardiovascular Care." Circulation. 2015; 132(suppl 2):S315–S367. doi: 10.1161/CIR.0000000000000252.

"Traveler's Checklist." Travel.State.Gov. https://travel.state.gov/content/travel/en/international-travel/before-you-go/travelers-checklist.html.

"Travelers' Diarrhea." CDC. https://wwwnc.cdc.gov/travel/page/travelers-diarrhea.

"Vaccines. Medicine. Advice." CDC. https://wwwnc.cdc.gov/travel.

"Your Health Abroad." Travel.State.Gov. https://travel.state.gov/content/travel/en/international-travel/before-you-go/your-health-abroad.html.

Yvette McQueen, MD. 2018. Travelpedia: A Quick Guide on How to Travel Efficiently, Healthy, and Safely.

Yvette McQueen, MD. "Jet Lag – Oops." Yvette McQueen, M.D. March 5, 2018. https://yvettemcqueenmd.com/blog-2/.

Yvette McQueen, MD. "Jet Lag – Oops." Yvette McQueen, M.D. March 5, 2018. https://yvettemcqueenmd.com/blog-2/.

Yvette McQueen, MD. "Post-Travel Illnesses." Yvette McQueen, M.D. May 3, 2018. https://yvettemcqueenmd.com/blog-2/.

Yvette McQueen, MD. "Is it food poisoning?" Yvette McQueen, M.D. May 22, 2018. https://yvettemcqueenmd.com/blog-2/.

Yvette McQueen, MD. "Wellness in Travel." Yvette McQueen, M.D. September 16, 2018. https://yvettemcqueenmd.com/blog-2/.

Yvette McQueen, MD. "Jet Lag – Oops." Yvette McQueen, M.D. March 5, 2018. https://yvettemcqueenmd.com/blog-2/.

Yvette McQueen, MD. "Traveling during the holidays." Yvette McQueen, M.D. November 30, 2018. https://yvettemcqueenmd.com/blog-2/.

Yvette McQueen, MD. "Summer feet – Pack your shower shoes." Yvette McQueen, M.D. June 23, 2020. https://yvettemcqueenmd.com/blog-2/.

Yvette McQueen, MD. "Travel Health: Pack Your Shower Shoes." Griots Republic. September 1, 2018. http://www.griotsrepublic.com/plantar-warts/.

About the Author

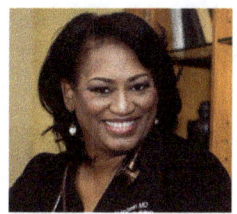

Yvette McQueen, MD, is an Emergency Medicine physician, travel doctor, instructor, speaker, entrepreneur, author, and consultant. She has traveled to over forty countries, serving both travelers and local residents, promoting health education, travel wellness, and disease prevention. Over the years, she has organized medical missions to Africa, performed hospital training in Rwanda and Tanzania, conducted wilderness emergency care training, taught internationally for the American Heart Association, and participated in international church missions.

As the CEO of MedQueen LLC, Dr. McQueen offers travel medicine, urgent care, and nutritional consultations via telemedicine to individuals, executives, and travel groups. As a locum tenens physician, she also travels across the United States and Caribbean, providing her services in hospitals' emergency departments.

Dr. McQueen obtained her medical degree from Medical College of Ohio in Toledo and completed her emergency medicine residency in Detroit, Michigan. Previous works include *Travelpedia* and *Inspiration in the Clouds*.

Learn more at www.yvettemcqueenmd.com

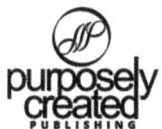

CREATING DISTINCTIVE BOOKS
WITH INTENTIONAL RESULTS

We're a collaborative group of creative masterminds with a mission to produce high-quality books to position you for monumental success in the marketplace.

Our professional team of writers, editors, designers, and marketing strategists work closely together to ensure that every detail of your book is a clear representation of the message in your writing.

Want to know more?
Write to us at info@publishyourgift.com
or call (888) 949-6228

Discover great books, exclusive offers, and more at
www.PublishYourGift.com

Connect with us on social media

@publishyourgift

www.ingramcontent.com/pod-product-compliance
Lightning Source LLC
Chambersburg PA
CBHW071113030426
42336CB00013BA/2068